Contents

High Blood Pressure Explained:

Natural, Effective, Drug-Free Treatment for the "Silent Killer"

By C.K. Murray

Similar works by C.K. Murray:

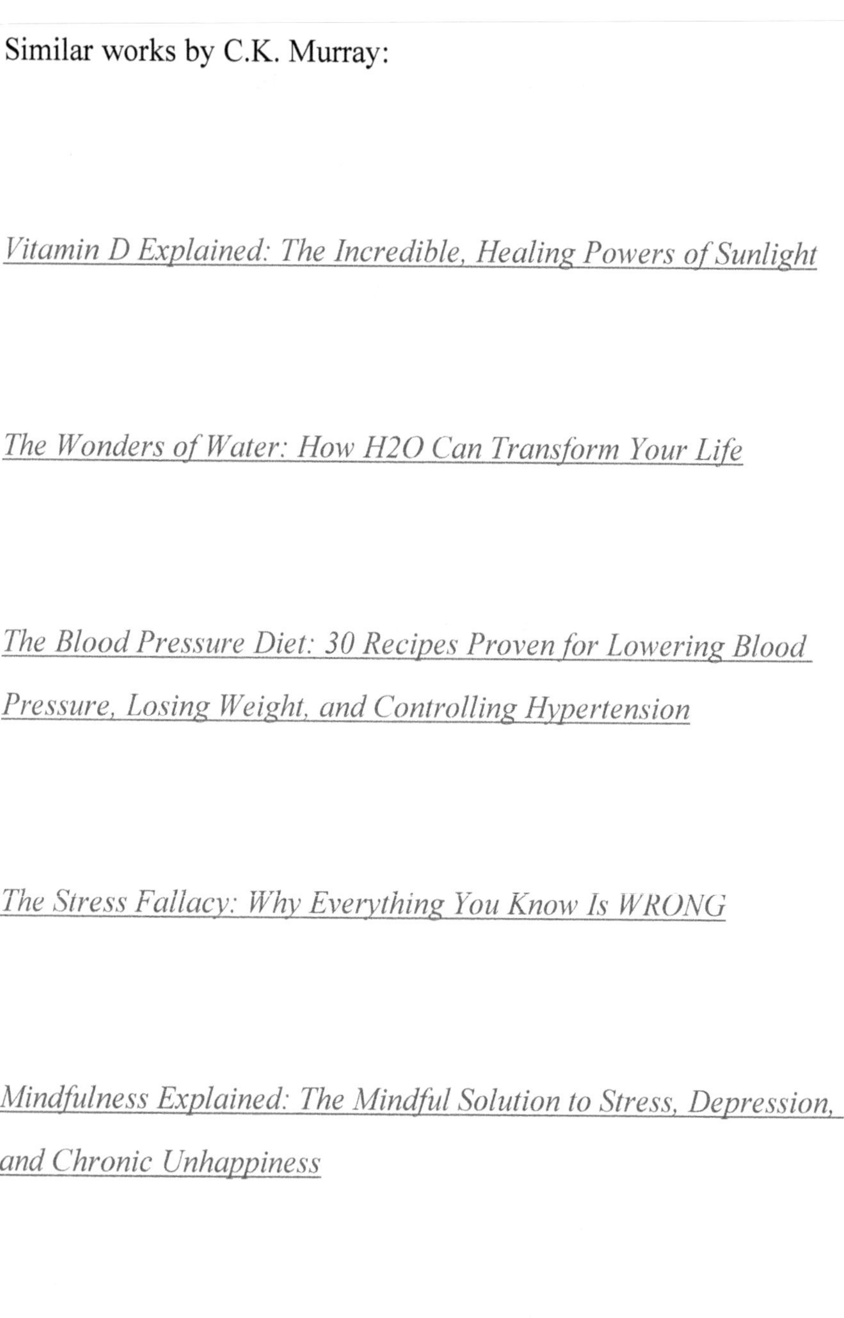

Vitamin D Explained: The Incredible, Healing Powers of Sunlight

The Wonders of Water: How H2O Can Transform Your Life

The Blood Pressure Diet: 30 Recipes Proven for Lowering Blood Pressure, Losing Weight, and Controlling Hypertension

The Stress Fallacy: Why Everything You Know Is WRONG

Mindfulness Explained: The Mindful Solution to Stress, Depression, and Chronic Unhappiness

Introduction to Blood Pressure

Blood is vital. Every second, it rushes through our arteries, our veins, our arterioles and capillaries, spanning the vast tract of the *impossibly* complex human circulatory system.

Although we all need blood pressure to live (assuming we're not bionic), that same blood pressure might be hurting us. Worse yet, it might be *killing* us. This is why high blood pressure, aka hypertension, has taken on the ominous title of "silent killer."

And it's easy to see why. Think about the function of blood in your body for a second. You don't need to be an M.D. to understand how important blood is. It's an indispensable part of the human creature, bringing good things (like nutrients) to our organs, muscles, and tendons, as well as bad things (like toxins).

When blood zips through our body with too much force, too much pressure, it begins to wear us away. Sure, our body naturally responds—but that doesn't mean the response is a good one. Over time, all this thumping and pumping of that vital red stuff starts to weaken our plumbing, causing all sorts of maladies—the worst of which might be a full-on explosion.

Ever seen a pipe burst?

In people with high blood pressure, the likelihood of a, shall we say, 'mishap' greatly increases. Moreover, the rate of long-term damage also increases. And even worse, most of us never even notice it! Unless you just finished an intense bout of cardio, chances are you're not consciously aware of your blood beating in your veins.

So what do we do?

Well, the first step is understanding exactly what makes blood pressure, *high* blood pressure. So let's cover the bases…

Know What to Look For! Subtle and Severe Symptoms of Hypertension

About 1 in 3 adults in the United States currently have high blood pressure. In medical terms, high blood pressure is called "hypertension" because it is literally an increased tension within our arteries. Blood pressure is directly determined by *the amount of blood your heart pumps* **vs.** *the amount of resistance to that blood pump* within the arteries.

Basically, if your arteries are too narrow, and the blood is pumping like crazy, your blood pressure is likely to be quite high. Of course, you're also likely to go about your business and have no idea. Again, this is why high blood pressure can be so serious, and deserves your attention.

Fortunately, there are known symptoms that can denote high blood pressure. *Un*fortunately, most of these symptoms do not manifest until hypertension has reached a dangerously high, if not life-threatening, level. This is a point known as 'hypertension crisis' and requires immediate medical attention. If you can't contact emergency medical services, get somebody to drive you to the hospital.

For those suffering a 'hypertension crisis,' the following **bold** symptoms may or may not occur. For those who have hypertension, but are *not* in crisis, the same symptoms may occur, including the other non-bold symptoms. The deciding factor in determining whether or not you or a loved one is suffering a 'hypertension crisis' is your reading: 180 or higher for your systolic pressure (top number) or 110 or higher for your diastolic pressure (bottom number).

The symptoms include:

- Dull headaches

- **Severe Headaches**

- **Nosebleeds**

- **Shortness of Breath**

- **Severe Anxiety**

- **Problems with your brain, such as memory loss, personality changes, concentration issues, irritability or progressive loss of consciousness (encephalopathy)**

- **Stroke**

- **Severe damage to the main artery (aortic dissection)**

- **Seizures in pregnant women (preeclampsia or eclampsia)**

- **Unstable chest pain (angina)**

- **Heart attack**

- **Sudden loss of kidney function (acute renal failure)**

- Dizzy Spells

- Facial Flushing

- Blood Spots in the Eyes

Again, if any of the above bold symptoms come on suddenly, it is important to seek medical attention. Many health practitioners may even *eliminate* high blood pressure as a potential cause, if other conditions are more likely. Still, it is wise not to mess around and simply 'ignore' the issue, especially when it's potentially lethal. Better safe than sorry, as they say.

Remember, high blood pressure can become very critical, very quickly. If you are at all unsure about yourself or somebody you know, and think high blood pressure is a mediating factor, do not hesitate to seek professional help. Also, be sure to education yourself as much as possible. Especially if high blood pressure runs in your family.

Going too long without controlling blood pressure may result in very serious problems to all areas of your body. Let's take a closer look:

Damage to the arteries

Good arteries are flexible, powerful and elastic. When healthy, their inner lining is smooth so that blood flows easily, which allows tissues and organs to receive vital nutrients. In people with hypertension, the increased pressure of blood flowing through the arteries eventually causes:

- ***Artery damage and narrowing***

High blood pressure hurts the cells of the arteries' inner lining. This makes artery walls thick and stiff, known as arteriosclerosis, or hardening of the arteries. Fats from one's diet enter the bloodstream, pass through the damaged cells and begin to start atherosclerosis.

These changes eventually block blood flow to the heart, kidneys, brain, arms and legs. This damage can then result in:

chest pain (angina),

heart attack,

heart failure,

kidney failure,

stroke,

blocked arteries in the legs or arms (peripheral artery disease),

eye damage,

and aneurysms.

- *Aneurysm*

Over time, the constant pressure of blood moving through weakened arteries may cause a portion of its wall to grow and form a bulge (aneurysm). An aneurysm can potentially rupture and cause lethal internal bleeding. Aneurysms can form in any artery throughout the body, but are most common in the largest artery, the aorta.

Damage to the heart

The heart is the body's pump. Uncontrolled high blood pressure can damage that pump in a number of ways, including:

- *Coronary artery disease*

This disease affects the arteries that supply blood to the heart. Arteries narrowed by coronary artery disease don't permit blood to flow well, and when blood can't flow easily to the heart, one can experience chest pain, a heart attack, or irregular heart rhythms (arrhythmias).

- *Enlarged left heart*

High blood pressure causes the heart to work harder than necessary in order to pump blood. This causes the left ventricle to thicken or stiffen, which limits the ventricle's ability to pump blood. This condition increases the likelihood of heart attack, heart failure and sudden cardiac death.

- ***Heart failure***

In the long-term, the pressure on the heart causes the muscle to weaken and work less efficiently. Eventually, the heart simply begins to wear out and fail. Damage from heart attacks only complicates this.

Damage to the brain

Just like the heart, the brain also depends on a good blood supply to work properly and persist. But high blood pressure can make this very difficult, causing:

- ***Transient ischemic attack (TIA)***

Also called a mini-stroke, a transient ischemic attack is a short, temporary disruption in the brain's blood supply. It's usually caused by atherosclerosis or a blood clot — both of which can come from hypertension. A transient ischemic attack may often precede a complete stroke.

- ***Stroke***

A stroke is what happens when a portion of the brain is deprived of oxygen and nutrients, resulting in dead brain cells. Uncontrolled high blood pressure can damage and weaken the brain's blood vessels, causing them to narrow, rupture or even leak. High blood pressure may contribute to blood clots in the arteries which also bring on a stroke.

- ***Dementia***

There are a number of reasons for dementia. One cause, vascular dementia, results from the narrowing and blockage of the arteries that supply blood to the brain. It can also result from strokes, traced back to high blood pressure.

- ***Mild cognitive impairment***

Mild cognitive impairment is a transition stage between normal deterioration associated with aging and the more sinister issues caused by Alzheimer's disease. Like dementia, it can result from blocked blood flow to the brain during periods of high blood pressure damage.

Damage to the kidneys

The kidneys filter waste and toxins from the bloodstream. High blood pressure can injure both the blood vessels in and leading to the kidneys, leading to several types of kidney disease (nephropathy). Having diabetes will only further complicate things.

- ***Kidney failure***

High blood pressure is a primary reason for kidney failure. It can damage both large arteries leading to the kidneys and tiny blood vessels (glomeruli) inside the kidneys. As a result, high levels of fluid and waste can accumulate. This can lead to the need for dialysis or kidney transplantation.

- ***Kidney scarring***

Glomerulosclerosis is a type of kidney damage caused by the scarring of glomeruli. The glomeruli are tiny blood vessels within the kidneys that filter fluid and waste, and when damaged, the glomeruli cannot filter correctly, leading to kidney failure.

- ***Kidney artery aneurysm***

When a bulge in an artery leading to the kidney occurs, it's known as a kidney (renal) artery aneurysm. Gradually, high blood pressure can cause an aneurysm — which can lead to lethal complications.

Damage to the eyes

- ***Eye blood vessel damage*** (retinopathy)

High blood pressure can damage the vessels that fuel the retina, causing retinopathy. This condition can lead to bleeding, blurred vision and complete loss of vision.

- ***Fluid buildup under the retina*** (choroidopathy)

This is a condition where fluid builds up under the retina because of a leaky blood vessel. Choroidopathy can result in scarring and distorted vision.

- ***Nerve damage*** (optic neuropathy)

In optic neuropathy, blocked blood flow damages the optic nerve. This can destroy nerve cells in the eyes, which can lead to bleeding within the eye as well as vision loss.

Sexual dysfunction

Like in all parts of the body, chronic high blood pressure damages the lining of the blood vessels and causes the arteries to harden and narrow (atherosclerosis), decreasing blood flow. When this happens in the penis, erectile dysfunction can result. This problem is fairly common, especially among men who do not control their high blood pressure.

Women may also experience sexual dysfunction as a result of high blood pressure. High blood pressure can reduce blood flow to the vagina, leading to a decrease in sexual desire or arousal, vaginal dryness, and trouble achieving orgasm. Improving arousal and lubrication may help this issue.

Miscellaneous dangers of high blood pressure

High blood pressure can also lead to:

- ***Bone loss***

High blood pressure can increase the amount of calcium that's in your urine, meaning that you lose urine at an excessive rate. This can lead to osteoporosis and an increased risk for broken bones.

- ***Sleep difficulties***

Obstructive sleep apnea is a condition where your throat muscles relax and cause snoring — and it occurs in more than half of those with high blood pressure. Furthermore, sleep deprivation that results from sleep apnea can boost the blood pressure.

- ***Metabolic syndrome***

This syndrome is caused by disorders in the body's metabolism, including increased waist circumference; high triglycerides; low high-density lipoprotein (HDL); high blood pressure; and high insulin levels.

Those with hypertension suffer other components of metabolic syndrome, which increases the risk of developing diabetes, heart disease or stroke.

Now that we have an idea of the symptoms and complications of high blood pressure, it is important to know what causes these problems. Truth be told, there are *many* causes of high blood pressure. And virtually *all* of them can be treated with lifestyle changes…

Where It Came From—The Numerous and Treatable Causes of Hypertension

Although we have a tendency to attribute much of the condition to genetics, hypertension is by no means out of our control. High blood pressure *can* be prevented or delayed by recognizing its causes.

Even so, as many as 95% of reported high blood pressure cases in the U.S have no certain etiology. In other words, for most cases, doctors cannot point to any one tangible cause. This type of hypertension is called 'essential hypertension.'

Although essential hypertension may be mysterious, it is certainly linked with many risk factors, and experts agree that reducing or eliminating these risk factors can often greatly reduce the chance of developing hypertension.

Some of the more important risk factors to consider are heredity, sex, age, and race. High blood pressure often runs in families and is more common among men than women. It is also more common among blacks, with blacks twice as likely as whites to develop high blood pressure. After the age of 65, black women have the highest incidence of high blood pressure.

Essential hypertension is also caused by salt intake. People in northern Japan eat more salt than anybody else, and show the highest incidence of high blood pressure. On the other hand, people who add no salt to their food show little to no signs of hypertension.

Other factors linked to essential hypertension include obesity; stress; diabetes; lack of potassium, magnesium, and calcium; lack of physical activity; and long-term alcohol use.

In cases where a direct cause is known for hypertension, the condition is called 'secondary hypertension.' Studies show that kidney disease, tumors, birth control pills, and pregnancy can all directly cause high blood pressure, as can medications that contract blood vessels.

So in review, the causes of hypertension include:

- Being overweight or obese

- Too much salt in the diet

- Too much alcohol consumption (more than 1 to 2 drinks per day)

- Smoking

- Lack of physical activity

- Stress

- Pregnancy

- Birth control

- Tumors

- Older age

- Family history of high blood pressure

- Chronic kidney disease

- Genetics

- Adrenal and thyroid disorders

With all of these factors, it may seem difficult to actually do anything about high blood pressure. The good thing is, with many factors come many solutions. Whether eating certain foods, avoiding others, learning relaxation techniques, exercising, boosting your emotional intelligence or simply changing your perspective, high blood pressure is definitely preventable and treatable.

EASY and NATURAL Strategies for Blood Pressure Reduction

Medication should never be the first step. The first step belongs to natural treatment, because natural treatment will not only cause fewer complications, but will also improve other areas of a person's life. Before even changing one's diet, one should consider the possibility of dealing with stress. Learning how best to harness stress is of vital importance.

When stressed, your body produces a spike of hormones. These hormones temporarily increase your blood pressure by forcing your heart to beat faster and your blood vessels to constrict. Because acute stress and certain extended periods of stress have actually been shown to be beneficial, one should not adopt the attitude that stress is generally bad. However, we should all understand that stress is perceptually-based. If we perceive things as uncontrollable, and our efforts as futile, we are unlikely to be happy. Moreover, our stress is likely to become unbearable.

When stress becomes so engrained, so all-controlling, we tend to lose ourselves. Instead of recognizing stressful events as springboards for self-improvement, we begin to lose our grasp. Instead of feeling good, we break down. The stress roots itself in our being, literally festering in our tightened muscles, wrapping around our arteries and constricting them.

When looking for ways to keep stress at levels that we can actively *harness*, we must remember our many options:

Rescheduling—If you feel like you have no time to unwind or do what you want, take a look at your schedule. Eliminate needless activities. Create a plan so you can use your stressful moments for when they matter—a desired creative pursuit, an important business day, an exciting but intimidating new date.

Exercise—Working out is an important part of healthy living. If you've already been diagnosed with high blood pressure, exercise not only reduces stress but can also reduce your systolic blood pressure anywhere from 5 to 10 millimeters of mercury (mm Hg). That's a big deal, and doesn't require a lot of time. Even just walking around the block can pay huge dividends. Not to mention, your mood will improve as a result of endorphins. And so will your weight!

Relaxation—Learn about biofeedback. Understand that you can consciously appraise your body's reactions to stress. You can learn to lower your blood pressure simply by recognizing what causes it to increase. You can change your thinking by addressing why something bothers you. Breathe to relax. Breathe deeply and slowly. Try yoga, try meditation. These activities can reduce your blood pressure as much as

5 millimeters of mercury (mm Hg). They have even been linked to gyrification, which researches believed causes cerebral cortex folding, and thus, improved neural processing. Basically, you'll feel better, be healthier, and you might even think better too!

And speaking of thinking, when changing your thinking, remember to consider why you feel the way you do:

- Does the intensity of my feelings correspond with the circumstances?

- Do I have more than one feeling that I'm dealing with?

- What are my interpretations?

- In what ways can I express myself?

- What are the effects of these expressions on me?

- What are the effects of these expressions on others?

- What conclusion am I seeking?

- What do I wish to do?

- Would it be better if I did nothing?

Feelings play a huge role in how we perceive our world. When you think negatively, you feel bad and this can manifest in your body. You may feel sore, tired, aching—and your internal organs and processes will mirror this. Your brain won't fire as cleanly, your arteries will constrict, and your organs won't work as efficiently.

Basically, your mind is your body, and your body is your mind. They are not separated by any stretch, and depend very closely upon one another for optimal functioning. Which is why we must, must, *must* watch how we fuel them. And *that* begins with what we put in our mouths…

18 AMAZING Foods for Reducing Hypertension

When it comes to changing our diets, the power is ours! Did you know that there are countless *amazing* foods out there rich with nutrients, vitamins, and a bunch of other mind and body-boosting goodies? The best part is, you don't have to have a lot of money to acquire these items. In fact, they are all widely available and affordable. Enjoying a heart-healthy diet is much easier than you think.

Take a look at the following great foods for lowering blood pressure, and learn to incorporate them into your diet. Dieticians may argue as to what constitutes a balanced meal, but ultimately the choice is yours. If you're not eating something from the list, try to make it part of your daily routine. Remember, the trick is not to overdo any one food group, as problems can also arise from extremity. Instead, try to mix and blend different combinations of these foods. You might just find the perfect recipe!

Bananas—These goodies are everywhere. Try to find some organic ones from a farmer's market or local producer. Even if you don't, supermarket 'nanas will do just fine. The great thing about bananas is that they are low in sodium, which is a leading precipitant of hypertension. They are also chock full of potassium, which can help low pressure by lowering the heart rate and protecting the muscles.

If you don't already, eat bananas in the whole. Or, if you prefer them in another form, put them in a fruit salad, cereal, and even grill or sauté them. There are plenty of ways to prepare the versatile banana.

White Potatoes—Like bananas, white potatoes such as the Idaho potato are rich in potassium. They are also very good for three other reasons. Firstly, they have little sodium, which is terrible for people with high blood pressure. Secondly, they are a good source of fiber, a critical part of every diet. And finally, white potatoes have no fat or cholesterol.

Although potatoes are sometimes thought to be unhealthy, this is largely a result of the way they are prepared. Dousing your potatoes with butter and salt will make them unhealthy. Instead, bake your potatoes and throw on an herb blend and/or some low-fat sour cream for a delicious and nutritious meal or side-meal.

Red Wine—Although too much alcohol increases one's risk of high blood pressure other health concerns, in moderation red wine soothes the arteries, diminishes blood sugar and lessens the risk of diabetes. Most experts define this as one five-ounce glass per day for women and up to two for men.

Wine contains ethyl alcohol (ethanol) and antioxidant polyphenols, such as resveratrol and procyanidins. Red wine, which contains 10 times the polyphenol content of white wine, is considered the healthiest for blood pressure. So drink up! Just not too much…

Fish—Like all foods, the fresher the better. Aside from being a great source of Omega Fats, fish is also laden with lean protein and Vitamin D. Vitamin D is crucial for a lot of things, but it also has been shown to lower blood pressure. Although we get Vitamin D from the sun, many of us don't get enough from food.

In order to prepare fish healthily, it's best to use just a light brushing of olive oil, and maybe some herbs. Baked or grilled for a few minutes, this recipe will guarantee an easy and tasty filet.

Broccoli—this green vegetable is another 'super-food.' It has awesome antioxidant and anti-inflammatory properties, and is packed full of fiber, calcium, potassium, magnesium, and vitamin C. All these nutrients work together to lower blood pressure.

A single cup of broccoli contains 200 percent of vitamin C for daily intake, and helps protect nitric oxide. Most people would do well to eat at least one serving a day. You can eat it raw with salsa or hummus, or steamed with olive oil and lemon. Or you can even juice it!

Dark Chocolate—Like wine, chocolate also contains polyphenols, a primary class of bioactive phytochemicals shown to protect against heart and vascular disease. A high concentration of flavonoids is also found in dark chocolate, which further promotes reduced blood pressure. Natural unsweetened cocoa powder has the highest concentration of flavonoids of all chocolates. For a delicious and healthy blend, make a chocolate banana cake. It contains both great foods for lowered blood pressure and will make you feel awesome!

Avocado—This green and nutritious food is packed full of potassium, vitamins, minerals, phytonutrients and monounsaturated fat. Fresh avocado makes a great substitute for mayonnaise or butter on sandwiches. Avocado can also be made into a delicious guacamole dip. Throw in some low-salt pita chips, quesadillas and/or tacos and you're set!

Lima Beans—These beans are probably not as widely eaten as other varieties, but they should be. They are actually higher in potassium than many of those varieties, as well as being great sources of fiber and protein.

Lima beans are best served by boiling them until tender in water. They can be eaten individually or as a complementary part of any vegetable broth. They can also be served cold and marinated, by themselves or in a salad.

Spinach—Spinach is one of those leafy greens that people either seem to love or hate. Either way, it's an incredibly healthy food. There are numerous benefits to eating spinach, such as its calcium content and low-sodium constitution. Not to mention, it is loaded with dietary fiber, iron, and Vitamins A and C. Basically, it's a "super-food."

Spinach is also great because it can be eaten a variety of ways. It can be cut up for salads, put into pasta, casseroles and other dishes. You can even throw it into a blender and make your own veggie smoothie. Regardless of your method, take advantage of spinach! It's awesome for you!

Yogurt—This is another great one. Studies show that calcium deficiency is a big contributor to hypertension, and with yogurt's super rich calcium content—about 1/3 an adult's recommended daily intake in one 6-ounce serving—this is the perfect solution.

Adults need calcium just like children, so eat up! Yogurt can be eaten by itself, and as a supplement to a smoothie. The beauty in yogurt is that it goes well with a lot of things. Healthy, tasty and versatile—what more do you need?

Blueberries—Again, blueberries contain those important natural compounds called flavonoids. They lower blood pressure, and taste good. They also serve as great alternatives to refined sugar by providing you a nice, short-term dosage of energy. You can eat blueberries by themselves, in cereal, in desserts—with virtually anything.

Oatmeal—Speaking of blueberries, oatmeal goes great with them! Oatmeal is that perfect high-fiber, low-fat, and low-sodium food the body needs for lowering blood pressure. Also, oatmeal is a great kickoff in the mornings.

Because many people find oatmeal to be bland, mix things up by throwing in some fruit, and maybe a dab of honey, and *voila*! This one's a no-brainer.

Sunflower Seeds (*Unsalted*)—Generally speaking, most nuts and legumes are very heart-healthy, assuming they aren't covered in salt. When it comes to sunflower seeds, they're extremely high in vitamin E, reaching 75 percent of your daily intake after just a handful.

Sunflower seeds are also full of folic acid and protein and fiber. Researchers have found that sunflower seeds release a peptide that inhibits the body's production of an enzyme known to raise blood pressure. Although the process is still not fully understood, the results are promising. Put down the salt and pick up the seeds!

Eggs—There is a misconception that eggs are not heart healthy. The truth is, past studies have shown that yolks *do not* raise heart disease risk, and moreover, recent studies reveal that egg whites actually help to reduce blood pressure. Although more research is required, eggs are a certain source of protein, vitamin D, and other healthy nutrients.

Beet juice—According to a study published in April 2013 in the American Heart Association Journal, people who drank about eight ounces of beetroot juice experienced a decrease in blood pressure of roughly 10 mm Hg. Beet juice contains nitrate, which turns into the gas nitric oxide, which then expands blood vessels and facilitates blood flow. A glass a day could help sustain healthy blood pressure.

Skim Milk—A cold glass of skim milk delivers both calcium and vitamin D, and has been shown to lower blood pressure by 3 to 10 percent in multiple studies. Research suggests that people with low levels of calcium are at greater risk of high blood pressure. The important thing to remember is to drink milk that has less fat. This is why skim milk is optimal.

Raisins—According to the American College of Cardiology's 61st Annual Scientific Session in 2012, consuming raisins three times a day may drastically reduce blood pressure. Besides containing more potassium than bananas, raisins are nice and sweet, without damaging the teeth. They also contain antioxidants and help fight against degeneration of the eyes. Furthermore, they boost bone density, combat anemia, and are high in fiber. Not to mention, they are a great source of natural sugar, providing a needed boost of energy when you need it most.

Oh, and did I mention raisins have been shown to suppress hunger between meals? So if you want a few snacks, make it happen. You can eat away guilt free without feeling like a glutton.

Celery—Doctors of Traditional Chinese Medicine (TCM) have recommended celery or celery roots to patients with high blood pressure for over a century. Now entering western medical practice, celery is highly touted for its powerful effects. Studies show that celery contains phytochemicals known as phthalides, which relax muscle tissue in the artery walls, thus allowing for increased blood flow.

Researchers state that eating four stalks of celery per day is adequate for reducing blood pressure. To spice up the flavor and gain some protein, try adding some unsalted peanut butter or almond butter. Both forms contain monounsaturated fat, which is great for the heart.

Of course, what you eat is only part of the equation. Drinking the right drinks is also important. Infused waters are extremely healthy due to their vitamin and nutrient distribution. Make sure to consume a healthy balance of liquids and foods. Coconut oil is a great substitute for fatty butters or over-processed margarines.

8 Foods that are TERRIBLE for Hypertension

Just as we can increase our consumption of certain foods to lower blood pressure, we can also *decrease* our consumption of certain foods to lower blood pressure. The following foods are widely considered terrible for those with high blood pressure, and will result in a variety of problems if not limited. *Especially* if not limited.

Salt—This one is always considered the main culprit when it comes to hypertension. The Dietary Guidelines for Americans suggests that people with hypertension or prehypertension limit their daily sodium intake to only 1,500 milligrams. Currently, the average American eats roughly 3,400 milligrams a day.

Research shows that more than 3/4 of the sodium you eat in a day comes from packaged foods, and not from the saltshaker. Some of these salty pre-packaged foods include deli meat, frozen pizza, canned soup, canned or bottled tomato products, and fruit and vegetable juices.

Deli meats—Speaking of salty foods, processed deli and lunch meats can be super bad for you. Because these meats are typically cured, seasoned, and preserved with salt, a single two-ounce serving of some lunchmeats could amount to over 600 milligrams of sodium. For the most part, stay away from processed foods. Especially cold cuts… even though they *are* delicious.

Sugar—Not only is excessive sugar linked to weight gain and obesity, but it also increases the likelihood of high blood pressure. Sugar, especially in sugar-sweetened drinks, has contributed to an increase in obesity in all people. The American Heart Association recommends that women limit added sugar intake to 6 teaspoons a day, and that men keep it near 9 teaspoons per day.

Alcohol—this little devil is in *a lot* of beverages. With alcohol, things can get a little tricky. Although small to moderate amounts of alcohol may lower your blood pressure, drinking too much can increase your blood pressure, even for people who only drink from time to time. Having more than three drinks in one sitting can cause a transient jump in blood pressure, and repeated drinking can lead to chronic high blood pressure.

Whole Wheat—In general, whole wheat is better. Whole wheat pasta, rice, bread, cereal, and other edibles can all reduce blood pressure. Make your oatmeal, rice, and pasta without salt in the cooking water, and you'll end up with 5 mg of sodium per serving.

Canned Goods—Get away from the habit of eating canned soups and broths. They are easy enough to make yourself as long as you have some water and time, and you can just as easily flavor them with vegetables, herbs, and spices at a low cost. Also, if you don't want to make your own, seek out low-sodium or no-salt-added versions of popular soups, broths, and vegetables. Also, you might want to can or freeze your own vegetables.

Biscuits—Refrigerated biscuit and crescent rolls contain trans fats, which are pretty bad news. According to the Harvard School of Public Health, trans fats are associated with an increased risk of high blood pressure in middle-aged and older women. Although labels might say that there are no trans fats, if the product contains hydrogenated oil in its ingredient list, it contains trans fats.

Instead, try whole grain bread or dinner rolls. Just be sure to check the ingredients labels!

Pizza—Meat-topped and plain cheese pizzas are full of unhealthy sodium. Given that salt is in the sauce, the crust, the cheese, and all the toppings like sausage, pizza is a great food if you're looking to jack up your blood pressure. As an alternative to cheese and meat pizza, ask for veggies instead.

Remember, the body needs a little bit of everything. Each of our constitutions are different, so each person needs to experiment with varying levels of healthy foods while avoiding the unhealthy foods that bring on trouble. Although high blood pressure is partially genetic, diet can *dramatically* affect its occurrence.

This is why medical experts and dieticians have come up with *Dietary Approaches to Stop Hypertension* (DASH). DASH is an eating plan full of everything that your body needs. These foods are overflowing with important nutrients like potassium, magnesium, calcium, fiber, and protein.

Because this diet has less salt and sugar than the typical American diet, it is a great plan for those willing to take serious, *natural* measures to lower blood pressure.

Creators of DASH give the following recommendations for a daily diet (based on 2,000 calories a day):

- *Grains: 7-8 daily servings (serving sizes: 1 slice of bread, 1/2 cup cooked rice or pasta, 1 ounce dry cereal)*

- *Vegetables: 4-5 daily servings (1 cup raw leafy greens, 1/2 cup cooked vegetable)*

- *Fruits: 4-5 daily servings (1 medium fruit, 1/2 cup fresh or frozen fruit, 1/4 cup dried fruit, 6 ounces fruit juice)*

- *Low-fat or fat-free dairy products: 2-3 daily servings (8 ounces milk, 1 cup yogurt, 1.5 ounces cheese)*

- *Lean meat, poultry, and fish: 2 or fewer servings a day (3 ounces cooked meat, poultry, or fish)*

- *Nuts, seeds, and legumes: 4-5 servings per week (1/3 cup nuts, 2 tablespoons seeds, 1/2 cup cooked dry beans or peas)*

- *Fats and oils: 2-3 daily servings (1 teaspoon vegetable oil or soft margarine, 1 tablespoon low-fat mayonnaise, 2 tablespoons light salad dressing)*

- *Sweets: less than 5 servings per week. (1 tablespoon sugar, jelly, or jam)*

The Fear Factor: Understanding "White Coat" Syndrome

By this point, you've realized that hypertension is no joke. And neither is understanding your reading. The problem is, there are a bunch of phony readings out there. Unless you are using a quality home product, the only way you can really know your true blood pressure is at your doctor's office.

And even this reading may sometimes vary. See, some people just don't like the doctor's office. Sure, doctors are there to ultimately help us, but certain people get nervous, really nervous, when at the doctor's. They feel unfamiliar; unsettled. They fear potential medical problems.

This can cause hypertension to spike.

When this spike occurs, we call it "white coat" syndrome, which comes from references to the white coats traditionally worn by doctors. On average, when your blood pressure is taken at home the top (systolic) number can be around 10mmHg lower than it would be if taken by a doctor and 5mmHg lower on the bottom (diastolic) number. For people with severe cases of white coat syndrome, these differences can be even greater. In fact, if you're super anxious, your systolic blood pressure can rise by as much as 30mmHg. This can make it more difficult for your doctor to get an accurate reading.

White coat hypertension refers to readings that are consistently 140/90mmHg or above *only* when in a medical setting. These blood pressure readings may be entirely normal when at home. Because of this, doctors will sometimes ask patients to take a few moments to relax before giving their reading.

Of course, for some people this just won't work. Some doctors may elect to prescribe 24-hour monitoring. In these cases, patients are given a small digital monitor to wear which then measures blood pressure automatically throughout day and night. Because the readings are stored in the device's memory, you can easily see your average, and thus *true*, blood pressure reading.

Know Your Numbers! How to Make Sense of Your Blood Pressure Reading

Once you've discovered your *true* blood pressure, it's time to know if you're in the 'danger zone.' This starts with understanding your reading. More specifically, knowing what both top and bottom numbers really mean.

Top number

The top number, which is also the higher of the two numbers, measures the pressure in the arteries when the heart beats (when the heart muscle contracts). This is called systolic.

Bottom number

The bottom number, which is also the lower of the two numbers, measures the pressure in the arteries between heartbeats (when the heart muscle is resting between beats and refilling with blood). This is called diastolic.

The American Heart Association recommends a blood pressure screening at your regular healthcare visit or once every 2 years, starting at the age of 20. This is, of course, if your blood pressure is less than 120/80 mm Hg. Although blood pressure can change depending upon posture, exercise, stress or sleep, it should normally be less than 120/80 mm Hg (less than 120 systolic AND less than 80 diastolic) for an adult age 20 or over.

If you want to take matters into your own hands and monitor your blood pressure regularly throughout the day, on your own terms, you have been careful. There are plenty of blood pressure monitors or 'readers' out there, and many of them are faulty, inconsistent, and/or simply cheap.

The number 1 doctor and pharmacist recommended brand is the Omron 7 Series. It's not cheap, at about $50, but it's definitely valid and reliable. For blood pressure, that's what matters.

If you're in the normal range, you're fine. If you're in the prehypertension stage, it's time to start taking measures to change your life. If you're in the other stages, you will want to make lifestyle changes as well as consultations with your physician. Just remember, before you take your blood pressure, try to avoid caffeine, cigarettes, and exercise for at least 30 minutes.

In the end, high blood pressure is not *the* end of the world. There are many things we can do before we reach a state of high blood pressure. It can be controlled, and it can be prevented. If we know what to look for, what to expect, and what to correct, we can all change our lives for the better.

So let's hold off on the medication just yet. Let's take a step back and make the changes in our lives that will make our lives healthier and happier. Hypertension may be called the 'silent killer,' but it doesn't have to be. That is, as long as we're listening…

***

A Special Note:

Thank you for reading "High Blood Pressure Explained: Natural, Effective, Drug-Free Treatment for the "Silent Killer." If you enjoyed this book and would like to read more like it, do not hesitate!

Other works by C.K. Murray:

      1.   *Mindfulness Explained: The Mindful Solution to Stress, Depression, and Chronic Unhappiness*

      2.   *Emotional Intelligence Explained: How to Master Emotional Intelligence and Unlock Your True Ability*

      3.   *The Confidence Cure: Your Definitive Guide to Overcoming Low Self-Esteem, Learning Self-Love and*